COMPLETE GUIDE TO BOWEL OBSTRUCTION

A Comprehensive Manual With Expert Insights, Diagnosis Techniques, Treatment Strategies, And Prevention Measures For Digestive Health Optimization

DEHART HAIRSTON

© [DEHART HAIRSTON], [2024]

All rights reserved. No part of this publication may be reproduced, distributed, or transmitted in any form or by any means, including photocopying, recording, or other electronic or mechanical methods, without the prior written permission of the publisher, except in the case of brief quotations embodied in critical reviews and certain other noncommercial uses permitted by copyright law.

DISCLAIMER

This book's content is only intended for general informative purposes. At the time of writing, the author has taken every precaution to guarantee that the material is correct and current. Nevertheless, the author disclaims all explicit and implicit representations and guarantees about the availability, appropriateness, correctness, completeness, and usefulness of the material on these pages.

Since the author is not a licensed medical practitioner, the material in this book shouldn't be interpreted as medical advice. Before making any modifications to their diet, exercise regimen, or medical treatment, readers are urged to speak with a licensed healthcare provider.

Moreover, the author has no connection to any of the businesses, organizations, or people that are discussed in this book. Any mentions of goods, services, businesses, or people are purely informative and do not indicate endorsement or suggestion.

This book's content is entirely dependent on the author's expertise, study, and comprehension of the topic. Despite having taken reasonable care to offer correct information, the author disclaims all liability for any mistakes or omissions in the material as well as for any losses, harm, or damages resulting from using the information.

It is recommended that readers use their own judgment and discretion when applying the knowledge in this book to their own situations. The use or implementation of any material in this book may result in unfavorable repercussions, directly or indirectly, for which the author assumes no liability.

By reading this book, you agree to release and hold the author harmless from any claims, losses, liabilities, costs, or expenditures resulting from or related to the use of the information you get from it.

Table of Contents

CHAPTER 1 11
- Understanding Bowel Obstruction 11
- What Is Bowel Obstruction? 11
- Causes Of Bowel Obstruction 11
- Types Of Bowel Obstruction 12

CHAPTER 2 15
- Signs And Symptoms 15
- Recognizing Symptoms Early 15
- Common Signs Of Bowel Obstruction 16
- When To Seek Medical Help 17

CHAPTER 3 19
- Diagnosis 19
- Medical History And Physical Examination 19
- Imaging Tests For Diagnosis 20
- Laboratory Tests And Other Diagnostic Procedures 22

CHAPTER 4 25
- Treatment Options 25
- Non-Surgical Treatments 25
- Surgical Interventions 26
- Lifestyle Changes And Home Remedies 28

CHAPTER 5 31
Complications 31
Potential Risks Of Bowel Obstruction 31
Long-Term Effects And Complications 32
Prevention Strategies 34
CHAPTER 6 37
Diet And Nutrition 37
Bowel-Friendly Foods 37
Foods To Avoid 39
Importance Of Hydration 40
CHAPTER 7 43
Recovery And Rehabilitation 43
Post-Treatment Care 43
Rehabilitation Exercises 45
Mental Health Support 47
CHAPTER 8 49
Coping Strategies 49
Coping With Chronic Bowel Obstruction 49
Support Groups And Resources 52
Tips For Managing Stress 54
CHAPTER 9 57

Future Outlook 57
Advances In Bowel Obstruction Treatment 57
Diagnostic Innovations 57
Minimal Invasive Interventions 58
Enhanced Surgical Techniques 59
Personalized Therapies 60
Biomarker Discovery 61
Targeted Therapies 62
Predictive Modeling 62
Regenerative Medicine 63
Hope For Patients And Families 63
CHAPTER 10 65
Living With Bowel Obstruction: Real Stories 65
Inspirational Stories Of Recovery 65
Advice From Survivors And Caregivers 66
CONCLUSION 69
THE END 72

ABOUT THIS BOOK

"Bowel Obstruction" is more than simply a book; it's a lifeline for everyone dealing with this ailment. Within its pages is a thorough handbook that unravels the complexity of bowel blockage, providing readers with information and methods critical to their well-being. Let me explain why this book is necessary.

First, Chapter 1, "Understanding Bowel Obstruction," provides readers with a thorough understanding of the illness, its causes, and the many manifestations. This underlying information is critical for bringing clarity and demystifying what may seem overwhelming.

Chapters 2–5 discuss detection, diagnosis, therapy, and complications. Recognizing symptoms early on, navigating diagnostic tests, and comprehending treatment choices are all critical steps toward successful management. Furthermore, information about possible hazards and preventative techniques provides readers with the skills they need to protect their health proactively.

Chapter 6 focuses on food and nutrition, emphasizing the need for sufficient sustenance in controlling intestinal blockage. From bowel-friendly meals to hydration necessities, this section provides a practical guide for making dietary changes to improve quality of life.

Chapter 7 focuses on recovery and rehabilitation, with an emphasis on post-treatment care and mental health. Readers are directed toward holistic recovery via the use of rehabilitation activities and mental health assistance.

"Coping Strategies" in Chapter 8 is a beacon of hope, giving practical assistance for dealing with the emotional and psychological obstacles of persistent intestinal blockage. Support groups and stress management methods help to build resilience in the face of hardship.

Looking forward to Chapter 9, "Future Outlook," readers are heartened by the advances achieved in therapy and continuing research. This area inspires hope and illuminates a route ahead for patients and families.

Finally, Chapter 10, "Living with Bowel Obstruction: Real Stories," provides a human touch by presenting genuine testimonies and inspiring stories. These accounts of perseverance and recovery serve as beacons of hope, reassuring readers that they are not alone on their path.

"Bowel Obstruction" is more than just a book; it's a road map to empowerment, providing priceless insights, practical advice, and unfailing support.

CHAPTER 1

Understanding Bowel Obstruction

What Is Bowel Obstruction?

Bowel obstruction is a severe medical disease in which a blockage prevents the usual movement of materials through the intestines. Consider traffic congestion on a freeway; similarly, a bowel obstruction causes a stoppage in the digestive tract, disturbing the smooth transit of food, fluids, and gas. This blockage may develop anywhere in the digestive system, from the small intestine to the large intestine (colon).

Causes Of Bowel Obstruction

Several reasons may cause bowel blockage. Adhesions, which are scar tissue bands that grow between intestinal loops, are a typical cause, often as a result of past abdominal surgery.

Other reasons include hernias, in which a portion of the intestine protrudes through a weak area in the abdominal wall, and tumors, which may physically obstruct the flow of intestinal contents. Bowel obstructions may also be caused by inflammatory disorders such as Crohn's disease or diverticulitis, which shorten or block the intestines. In addition, some disorders, such as volvulus, in which the intestine twists on itself, and intussusception, in which one segment of the intestine telescopes into another, may cause blockage.

Types Of Bowel Obstruction

Bowel blockages are separated into two types: mechanical and functional. Mechanical blockages happen when there is a physical blockage in the gut, such as a tumor or a hernia. Functional blockages, on the other hand, arise when the intestine's muscles fail to move contents forward in the absence of a physical blockage.

This may occur as a result of nerve or muscle disorders, such as paralytic ileus or pseudo-obstruction.

Mechanical obstacles are further classified according to the location of the blockage. Adhesions and hernias are common causes of minor bowel blockages. Large intestinal blockages in the colon are often caused by tumors, diverticulitis, or volvulus. Understanding the kind of blockage is critical for selecting the best treatment plan.

Each form of blockage causes a unique combination of symptoms and problems, ranging from stomach discomfort and bloating to nausea, vomiting, and constipation. Early detection and treatment of bowel obstruction is critical to avoiding significant consequences such as bowel ischemia (lack of blood supply to the intestine), perforation (tear in the intestinal wall), and sepsis (infection spreading via the bloodstream).

Individuals who understand the fundamentals of bowel blockage, including its causes and kinds, may better detect the signs and symptoms, seek prompt medical assistance, and collaborate with healthcare providers to establish an effective treatment strategy.

CHAPTER 2

Signs And Symptoms

Recognizing Symptoms Early

When it comes to intestinal blockage, early detection of symptoms is critical for timely medical action. Understanding the symptoms might help people seek care promptly, thereby averting problems and alleviating suffering. It is important to be watchful and detect any changes in your bowel habits or stomach pain.

Abdominal discomfort is an important symptom to be aware of. This pain often begins as cramping or discomfort in the abdomen, but it may soon worsen and become severe. The position of the discomfort varies depending on the underlying reason for the blockage, however, it is usually at the belly button or lower abdomen.

Pay attention to the kind of pain, since it might be acute, stabbing, or cramp-like.

Along with the discomfort, you may suffer bloating and a feeling of fullness in your belly. Bloating may make you feel as if your stomach is bloated or bulging. You may also notice changes in your bowel motions, such as constipation or diarrhea, depending on the kind of blockage.

Common Signs Of Bowel Obstruction

Bowel blockage may show in a variety of ways, and understanding the main symptoms can help you take proper action. Vomiting is a common symptom, especially when it persists and gets severe. The vomit may include partly digested food or bile, and in extreme situations, it might smell like feces or even contain blood.

Another distinguishing feature is the inability to pass gas or have a bowel movement. This happens when a blockage inhibits the usual transit of feces and gas through the gut. As a consequence, you may get progressively constipated or notice a total stop of bowel motions.

In certain situations, bowel blockage may cause fecal impaction, which occurs when tough feces deposits in the intestines, further restricting the channel. This might result in additional symptoms such as rectal soreness, liquid stool or mucus leaking, and the sensation of incomplete evacuation after bowel movements.

When To Seek Medical Help

Knowing when to seek medical attention is critical when coping with symptoms of intestinal blockage. If you have chronic stomach discomfort that develops over time or is accompanied by vomiting, you should seek medical assistance immediately. Furthermore, if you detect any unexpected changes in your bowel habits, such as severe constipation or diarrhea, particularly if they are accompanied by abdominal distension or bloating, you should see a healthcare practitioner right once.

Other warning flags include being unable to pass gas or have a bowel movement for a lengthy period, as well as indicators of dehydration such as dry lips, reduced urine production, or dizziness. These symptoms might signal a more serious blockage or consequences, such as intestinal perforation, necessitating immediate medical attention.

If you're unclear if your symptoms need medical treatment, it's best to err on the side of caution and see a healthcare expert. Early management may reduce complications and improve outcomes in instances of intestinal blockage.

CHAPTER 3

Diagnosis

Medical History And Physical Examination

When it comes to identifying intestinal blockage, medical history, and physical examination are crucial. Your doctor will begin by collecting a thorough medical history, including questions about your symptoms, medical problems, and any prior operations or treatments you have had. This information assists in determining probable causes and assessing the severity of your ailment.

During the physical exam, your doctor will check for particular indicators of intestinal blockage. They may palpate your abdomen to check for pain, distention, or abnormal lumps. Bowel sounds are also evaluated; diminished or nonexistent noises may suggest an obstruction.

Other physical symptoms, such as abdominal stiffness or guarding, may also be present, suggesting a more serious blockage.

In addition, your doctor may ask about your bowel habits, such as changes in frequency, consistency, or the presence of blood in your stool. These characteristics may give further information about the kind and location of the impediment. Overall, the medical history and physical examination are critical beginning stages in the diagnostic process, guiding further investigations and treatment options.

Imaging Tests For Diagnosis

Imaging investigations are critical in verifying the diagnosis of intestinal blockage and determining the underlying cause. Various imaging techniques may be employed, depending on the presumed source and severity of the blockage.

Abdominal X-rays are a regularly used imaging tool. These may indicate indicators of intestinal blockage, such as dilated bowel loops, increased air-fluid levels, and gas collection. X-rays are rapid and easy to get, making them an invaluable tool in the early detection of suspected intestinal blockage.

In addition to X-rays, computed tomography (CT) scans are often used to get more comprehensive pictures of the abdomen and pelvis. CT scans can correctly determine the location and source of the blockage, as well as any consequences such as intestinal perforation or ischemia. They are especially beneficial in circumstances when the diagnosis is ambiguous or surgical intervention is being considered.

Ultrasound imaging may also be employed in certain instances. While ultrasonography is less usually used to diagnose intestinal blockage, it may be useful, particularly in pediatric or pregnant patients, since it does not need radiation exposure. Ultrasound may identify characteristics indicative of blockage, such as dilated bowel loops and fluid collection, although it may be less sensitive than CT in certain cases.

Overall, imaging studies are useful in the diagnosis of intestinal blockage because they provide precise anatomical information that informs treatment options and helps determine the severity of the illness.

Laboratory Tests And Other Diagnostic Procedures

In addition to imaging studies, intestinal blockage may be diagnosed using a variety of laboratory testing and diagnostic methods.

Blood tests are frequently conducted to look for evidence of infection, electrolyte abnormalities, and dehydration, which are all typical consequences of intestinal blockage. Increased white blood cell count and aberrant electrolyte values, such as potassium and sodium, may indicate the existence of a blockage and aid in therapy.

Endoscopic techniques may be used when the reason for a blockage is unknown or more information is required. Colonoscopy or upper endoscopy (esophagogastroduodenoscopy) may be seen within the gastrointestinal system and detect structural abnormalities or blockages. These procedures are especially effective when there is a possibility of inflammatory bowel disease, tumors, or strictures causing the blockage.

Furthermore, contrast investigations such as barium enema or small bowel follow-through may be used to assess the structure and function of the intestines. In these tests, contrast material is ingested or administered and visible on X-rays or fluoroscopy, enabling the discovery of strictures, tumors, or narrowing regions that may be causing the blockage.

In conclusion, laboratory testing and diagnostic procedures supplement imaging investigations in the diagnosis of intestinal blockage by giving additional information about the underlying cause and contributing variables. By combining various diagnostic methods, healthcare practitioners may properly identify the intestinal blockage and provide a treatment plan that is personalized to the specific patient's requirements.

CHAPTER 4

Treatment Options

Non-Surgical Treatments

Non-surgical therapies are often used as the first line of defense for intestinal blockage. These techniques try to relieve symptoms and help the gut restore normal function without requiring surgery. One of the key approaches is bowel rest, in which the patient refrains from eating or drinking anything orally to enable the intestines to recover. During this period, fluids and nutrients may be delivered intravenously to keep the patient hydrated and fed.

The use of drugs is also an important element of nonsurgical therapy. Pain medications may be used to reduce discomfort, antiemetics to control nausea and vomiting, and antibiotics to prevent or cure infections.

In addition, laxatives or enemas may be administered to assist remove obstructions and encourage bowel movement.

In certain circumstances, physicians may also propose using a nasogastric tube. This tiny tube is placed via the nose and into the stomach to decompress the colon and remove excess gas and fluids. Nasogastric suction may assist in alleviating abdominal distension and lessen pressure on the blocked bowel, hence alleviating symptoms.

Surgical Interventions

When non-surgical therapies fail to relieve the intestinal blockage or there are indicators of consequences such as intestine perforation or tissue death, surgery may be required. The kind of surgery performed depends on the underlying reason and degree of the blockage.

One typical surgical technique for intestinal blockage is bowel resection. During this procedure, the blocked or damaged section of the intestine is removed, and the healthy ends are rejoined. This promotes the regular movement of digestive materials through the gut.

If the blockage is caused by scar tissue or adhesions, surgeons may employ a treatment known as adhesiolysis. Cutting or breaking up the scar tissue frees the intestine and allows it to operate correctly. A temporary stoma may be constructed to direct the passage of feces away from the damaged region while it recovers.

In more severe circumstances, such as extensive tissue injury or a fully clogged intestine, emergent surgery may be necessary. This may include bypassing the blocked section of the bowel or performing an ostomy, in which a part of the intestine is introduced through the abdominal wall to form a stoma for waste removal.

Lifestyle Changes And Home Remedies

In addition to medical therapies, lifestyle adjustments, and home remedies may help manage and prevent intestinal blockage. One of the most crucial components is to eat healthily and remain hydrated. A high-fiber diet rich in fruits, vegetables, and whole grains may help encourage regular bowel movements and lower the risk of constipation, which can lead to blockage.

Staying physically active might also assist in keeping the digestive system running properly. Regular exercise increases bowel motility and may help reduce the accumulation of gas and stool in the intestines. Furthermore, stress management strategies such as meditation or yoga may help minimize the risk of stomach pain and digestive disorders.

Individuals who are prone to repeated bowel blockages or have underlying diseases such as Crohn's disease or diverticulitis should work closely with a healthcare physician to build a specific treatment strategy. This may need frequent monitoring, prescription adjustments, and dietary changes customized to individual requirements and preferences.

In conclusion, although intestinal blockage is a difficult disease to manage, there are many therapeutic options available, ranging from non-surgical therapies to surgical operations. Individuals who combine medical treatments with lifestyle adjustments and home cures may successfully control their symptoms and enhance their quality of life.

CHAPTER 5

Complications

Potential Risks Of Bowel Obstruction

Bowel blockage may provide a variety of health hazards, ranging from pain to serious consequences requiring emergency medical intervention. The greatest danger associated with intestinal obstruction is the disruption of normal bowel function, which results in the collection of gas, fluids, and feces above the blockage. This accumulation may lead to severe stomach discomfort, bloating, and vomiting. If left untreated, the blockage pressure may cause tissue damage and even intestinal rupture, resulting in life-threatening infections and sepsis.

Another risk of intestinal blockage is dehydration. When the gut is obstructed, fluids cannot move properly, causing dehydration over time.

Dehydration may exacerbate symptoms including weakness, dizziness, and disorientation, necessitating IV fluids to restore normal hydration levels.

Furthermore, bowel blockage raises the risk of intestinal ischemia, which occurs when the blood supply to the gut is reduced. Reduced blood flow deprives the bowel of oxygen and essential nutrients, causing tissue damage and, in extreme instances, gangrene. Intestinal ischemia is a medical emergency that needs immediate treatment to avoid catastrophic consequences.

Long-Term Effects And Complications

Bowel blockage, if left untreated or delayed, may cause a variety of long-term repercussions and difficulties. One of the most serious long-term consequences is intestinal necrosis, which happens when a prolonged absence of blood supply causes tissue death in the gut. Bowel necrosis may result in severe stomach discomfort, fever, and infection, necessitating immediate surgery to remove the affected part of the intestine.

Chronic intestinal blockage may cause malnutrition and weight loss. When the gut is partly or obstructed, nutritional absorption is hindered, leading to vitamin and mineral shortages. This may deplete the immune system, impede wound healing, and contribute to general bad health.

Furthermore, repeated occurrences of intestinal blockage may result in the creation of scar tissue in the gut, known as adhesions. Adhesions may further constrict the intestinal lumen, raising the possibility of future blockages and complicating surgical procedures. To avoid problems and enhance quality of life, chronic bowel obstruction treatment may include dietary changes, medicines, and surgical treatments.

Prevention Strategies

While certain causes of bowel blockage, such as adhesions or certain congenital abnormalities, cannot be avoided, people may make efforts to lower their chances of acquiring the disease. One key preventative method is to eat a fiber-rich diet and remain hydrated. Adequate fiber consumption promotes regular bowel movements and prevents constipation, which may lead to intestinal blockage.

Furthermore, avoid habits that raise the likelihood of intestinal obstructions, such as swallowing big items, eating difficult-to-digest meals, or disregarding gastrointestinal symptoms. Prompt medical assistance should be sought if you have persistent stomach discomfort, bloating, or changes in bowel habits, as early detection and treatment may help avoid consequences from bowel blockage.

In situations when bowel blockage is caused by underlying medical disorders such as Crohn's disease or colon cancer, successfully controlling these illnesses may help prevent the obstruction from recurring. Depending on the situation, this might include medication, lifestyle changes, or surgical intervention.

Overall, a proactive approach to digestive health, along with early detection and treatment of symptoms, is critical for avoiding the problems of bowel blockage and sustaining overall health.

CHAPTER 6

Diet And Nutrition

Bowel-Friendly Foods

When dealing with intestinal blockage, selecting the proper meals is critical for reducing symptoms and promoting healing. Bowel-friendly meals are simple to digest, soft on the digestive system, and assist in avoiding future difficulties. These meals are often lacking in fiber and fat, making them difficult to digest during blockage.

One of the most common types of bowel-friendly diets is readily digested carbs. These include white rice, bread, spaghetti, and crackers. These carbs give energy while placing little burden on the digestive system. Cooked fruits and vegetables without skins or seeds are also advised since they are softer and simpler to digest than raw ones.

Lean proteins are another essential component of a bowel-friendly diet. Choose leaner meats like chicken, turkey, and fish, which are simpler to stomach than fatty portions. Eggs are also a fantastic source of protein and may be cooked in a variety of ways to suit different tastes.

Dairy products may be consumed in moderation, however, low-fat ones are vital to prevent excessive fat consumption. Plain yogurt, skim milk, and low-fat cheese are good options for those who have intestinal obstructions. These dairy products give calcium and protein without causing intestinal pain.

Including modest, regular meals is essential for controlling intestinal blockage symptoms. Eating smaller amounts throughout the day is less taxing on the digestive system than eating big meals. Furthermore, chewing food carefully and eating slowly may assist with digestion and lower the chance of difficulties.

Foods To Avoid

While certain meals are useful to people with intestinal blockage, others might worsen symptoms and should be avoided. High-fiber meals are often difficult for the intestines to digest during blockage, which may exacerbate symptoms like stomach discomfort and bloating.

Insoluble fiber-rich foods, such as whole grains, nuts, seeds, and raw fruits and vegetables, should be reduced or avoided completely. These foods bulk up the stool, which increases the risk of intestinal obstruction or worsens existing obstructions.

Fatty and oily meals should also be avoided since they are difficult for the body to digest and may worsen symptoms like nausea and vomiting. Fried meals, fatty cuts of meat, and high-fat dairy items should be avoided in the diet of people with intestinal blockage.

Foods that produce gas may cause stomach pain and bloating, exacerbating intestinal obstruction symptoms. Carbonated drinks, legumes, cruciferous vegetables (such as broccoli and cabbage), and certain fruits (such as apples and pears) are all known to cause gas and should be taken in moderation.

Caffeine and alcohol may have a laxative impact on the body, exacerbating diarrhea in those with intestinal blockage. These drugs should be limited or avoided to avoid future issues and enhance overall digestive health.

Importance Of Hydration

Staying hydrated is critical for people with intestinal blockage because it prevents dehydration and supports digestive function. When the intestines get obstructed, fluid may not flow through the digestive tract as effectively, raising the risk of dehydration.

Drinking enough water throughout the day helps keep the digestive system running smoothly and avoids difficulties like constipation. Aim to drink at least eight glasses of water every day, and more if you have diarrhea or vomiting.

In addition to water, electrolyte-rich fluids like sports drinks or oral rehydration treatments may assist restore fluids and electrolytes lost during intestinal blockage. These drinks include important minerals like sodium, potassium, and chloride, which are required for fluid equilibrium in the body.

Individuals with intestinal blockage should avoid dehydrating substances such as caffeine and alcohol. These drinks might cause more fluid loss and dehydration, exacerbating symptoms and complicating recovery.

To summarize, eating a colon-friendly diet and keeping hydrated are critical components of controlling intestinal obstructions. Individuals may maintain digestive health and help recovery from blockage by consuming the correct meals and drinks while avoiding those that might aggravate symptoms.

CHAPTER 7

Recovery And Rehabilitation

Post-Treatment Care

After receiving treatment for bowel blockage, whether by surgery or other medical procedures, it is critical to emphasize post-treatment care to ensure a smooth recovery. Post-treatment care includes wound care, pain management, dietary changes, and monitoring for problems.

First and foremost, carefully follow your healthcare provider's wound-care recommendations. Keeping the surgery site clean and dry is critical to avoiding infections. Change dressings as directed and contact your healthcare practitioner promptly if you see any indications of infection, such as increased redness, swelling, or discharge.

Pain management is another important component of post-treatment care. Your doctor will prescribe pain relievers to help you feel better throughout the healing process. It is critical to take these drugs exactly as recommended and to immediately express any concerns or changes in pain levels to your healthcare provider.

Dietary changes may be required after therapy for intestinal blockage. Your healthcare professional may prescribe a particular diet to follow throughout the recovery period, such as starting with a low-fiber or clear liquid diet and progressively progressing to solid meals as tolerated. It is critical to follow these dietary rules to prevent worsening symptoms and assist in the healing process.

Furthermore, careful monitoring for indicators of problems is essential throughout the post-treatment era. Keep an eye out for symptoms like persistent stomach discomfort, fever, nausea, vomiting, or changes in bowel habits, since these might suggest a serious problem that requires medical treatment. If you have any concerns or questions concerning the status of your recuperation, please contact your healthcare practitioner.

Rehabilitation Exercises

Rehabilitation activities are essential for recovering strength, mobility, and function after bowel blockage therapy, especially if surgery is required. These exercises attempt to enhance muscle tone, flexibility, and general physical fitness, allowing for a speedier recovery and lowering the chance of problems.

Depending on your exact circumstances and the scope of your therapy, your healthcare practitioner or physical therapist may prescribe exercises that are suited to your requirements. These exercises may include mild stretching, range-of-motion exercises, and focused abdominal muscle strengthening.

It is important to undertake rehabilitation activities under the supervision of a healthcare expert to guarantee safety and efficacy. Begin with mild exercises, gradually increasing in intensity and length as tolerated. Listen to your body and don't push yourself too hard, particularly during the early phases of healing.

Consistency is essential when it comes to rehabilitation activities. Aim to include these workouts in your everyday practice, gradually increasing your strength and mobility. Remember that rehabilitation is a lengthy process, and patience is required for best results.

In addition to physical therapy, do not underestimate the need for mental health care throughout the healing process.

Coping with a physical issue, such as bowel blockage, and going through treatment may hurt your mental well-being. It is natural to feel a variety of emotions, including worry, irritation, and dread.

Mental Health Support

Seeking mental health care will help you cope with the emotional obstacles of bowel blockage therapy. This assistance may take many forms, including therapy, counseling, support groups, or just talking to trustworthy friends and family about your thoughts and worries.

Therapy or counseling may provide a secure environment in which to explore and process your emotions, acquire coping methods, and build resilience in the face of hardship. A mental health expert can provide direction and support targeted to your specific requirements, assisting you in navigating the ups and downs of the recovery process.

Support groups may also be useful for connecting with others who have had similar issues. Sharing experiences, ideas, and encouragement with people who understand what you're going through may help you feel validated and supported. Online forums and social media groups may be great places to locate supportive communities.

Remember that it's normal to seek assistance when you need it, and you don't have to face the difficulties of rehabilitation alone. Contact your healthcare team, loved ones, or mental health specialists for assistance anytime you need it. Taking care of your emotional health is equally as essential as taking care of your physical health throughout the healing period.

CHAPTER 8

Coping Strategies

Coping With Chronic Bowel Obstruction

Living with persistent intestinal blockage may pose considerable physical and mental concerns. Coping methods are essential for controlling the disease and enhancing quality of life. Education is an important coping tool; knowing the nature of bowel blockage, its causes, symptoms, and treatment choices allows people to make educated decisions about their health.

Acceptance is another important component of dealing with persistent intestinal blockage. Accepting the condition does not imply surrender; rather, it entails accepting its existence and learning to adapt to its restrictions while still leading a full life.

This mentality adjustment might help people concentrate on what they can control rather than what they can't.

Building a solid support network is essential for dealing with persistent intestinal blockage. This network might include family members, friends, healthcare providers, and support groups. Surrounding oneself with understanding and caring people may provide emotional support, practical aid, and encouragement during difficult times.

Maintaining a healthy lifestyle is critical for treating persistent intestinal blockage. This involves eating a well-balanced diet high in fiber, keeping hydrated, and participating in frequent physical exercise. Furthermore, avoiding triggers, such as foods or activities that aggravate symptoms, may help reduce pain and prevent flare-ups.

Self-care is essential for those living with persistent intestinal blockage. This might include deep breathing exercises, meditation, or yoga to relieve stress and increase general well-being. It's also critical to prioritize sleep and rest, since exhaustion may exacerbate symptoms and impair everyday performance.

Seeking expert aid when required is another important component of dealing with persistent intestinal blockage. This may include talking with healthcare specialists to explore treatment choices, successfully managing pain and suffering, and treating any psychological or emotional issues related to the disease.

Overall, dealing with persistent bowel obstruction requires a multimodal strategy that includes knowledge, acceptance, support, lifestyle changes, self-care, and professional assistance. Individuals who follow these coping skills may better manage their disease and improve their overall quality of life.

Support Groups And Resources

Support groups may be excellent tools for those who have bowel blockage. These organizations provide a secure and accepting atmosphere in which members may discuss their experiences, exchange information, and give emotional support to one another. Participating in a support group may help people feel less alienated and more empowered to manage their disease efficiently.

Individuals may also interact with others who are dealing with similar intestinal blockage issues via online forums and social media platforms. These virtual communities provide a handy option to obtain assistance and information from the comfort of one's own home, regardless of geographical location.

In addition to peer support, people living with bowel blockage have access to a variety of options. These resources may include instructional materials, online articles, books, and credible websites that provide information about the ailment, treatment alternatives, and coping methods.

Individuals with intestinal blockage might benefit from the expertise of healthcare experts such as physicians, nurses, and allied health workers. These experts may give tailored advice, answer questions, and provide recommendations to other specialists or services as required.

Individuals must investigate various support groups and services to determine which ones best match their needs and preferences. Whether seeking in-person or online assistance, interacting with others and finding accurate information may help people negotiate the obstacles of living with bowel blockage more efficiently.

Tips For Managing Stress

Stress management is critical for those living with bowel blockage since it may increase symptoms and have a negative influence on overall health. Fortunately, people may use a variety of ways to decrease stress and increase relaxation.

Deep breathing exercises are an efficient stress-management method. Deep breathing consists of taking slow, deep breaths via the nose, filling the lungs with air, and then slowly expelling through the mouth. This technique may trigger the body's relaxation response, resulting in a sensation of serenity and contentment.

Mindfulness meditation is another effective stress-management technique. This technique entails paying attention to the present moment without judgment and letting ideas and sensations pass without getting attached to them. Mindfulness meditation has been demonstrated to lower stress, worry, and despair, making it an effective coping method for those living with intestinal blockage.

Regular physical exercise may also assist in reducing stress and enhance general health. Exercise causes the brain to produce endorphins, which function as natural mood boosters, increasing sensations of enjoyment and relaxation. Finding enjoyable ways to stay active, whether through walking, yoga, or participating in a favorite sport, can have a significant impact on stress management.

In addition to these techniques, individuals should prioritize self-care activities that promote relaxation and rejuvenation. This could include finding time for hobbies, spending quality time with loved ones, getting enough sleep, and practicing good sleep hygiene.

Finally, seeking professional help when needed is critical for effective stress management. Therapists and counselors can offer support, guidance, and coping strategies that are tailored to the individual's needs and circumstances.

Individuals with bowel obstruction can improve their overall well-being and cope with the challenges of their condition by incorporating these stress-management tips into their daily routines.

CHAPTER 9

Future Outlook

Advances In Bowel Obstruction Treatment

In recent years, significant advances in bowel obstruction treatment have been made, providing patients with new hope and better outcomes. These advancements affect various aspects of care, such as diagnosis, management, and surgical procedures. With the integration of cutting-edge technologies and innovative approaches, healthcare professionals are better equipped than ever to effectively treat bowel obstruction.

Diagnostic Innovations

Diagnostic techniques for bowel obstruction have advanced significantly. Traditional methods such as X-rays and CT scans are still useful, but newer modalities such as magnetic resonance imaging

(MRI) and ultrasound are gaining popularity. These advanced imaging technologies enable more precise and detailed visualization of the bowel, facilitating early detection and localization of obstructions. Furthermore, emerging biomarkers and molecular imaging agents show promise in improving diagnostic accuracy and guiding personalized treatment strategies.

Minimal Invasive Interventions

Minimally invasive procedures have transformed the treatment of bowel obstruction, providing numerous advantages over traditional open surgery. Laparoscopy and robotic-assisted surgery allow surgeons to access the affected area through small incisions, resulting in less postoperative pain, shorter hospital stays, and faster recovery times. These approaches are especially beneficial for frail or elderly patients who may not tolerate lengthy surgical procedures well. Furthermore, advances in endoscopic therapies, such as stent placement and balloon dilation, offer minimally invasive options for relieving obstructions and restoring bowel function without requiring major surgery.

Enhanced Surgical Techniques

Advances in surgical techniques have also helped to improve the outcomes of bowel obstruction treatment. Improved understanding of bowel physiology, combined with refined surgical approaches, has resulted in more targeted and effective interventions. Surgeons now have access to advanced tools and instruments that allow for precise tissue dissection, vascular preservation, and reconstruction, reducing intraoperative complications and improving functional outcomes. Furthermore, the use of intraoperative imaging modalities such as fluorescence-guided surgery improves surgical accuracy while decreasing the risk of complications, paving the way for safer and more successful procedures.

Personalized Therapies

The era of personalized medicine is transforming the landscape of bowel obstruction treatment, ushering in a new era of tailored therapies based on unique patient characteristics and disease profiles. Advances in genetics, molecular biology, and pharmacogenomics have shed light on the underlying mechanisms of bowel obstruction and identified potential therapeutic targets. Using this knowledge, healthcare providers can create personalized treatment plans that maximize efficacy while minimizing side effects. From targeted drug therapies to individualized surgical approaches, personalized medicine promises better outcomes and a higher quality of life for patients with bowel obstruction.

Research & Innovation

The field of bowel obstruction remains a fertile ground for research and innovation, with ongoing efforts to address unmet clinical needs and raise the standard of care. Researchers and clinicians around the world are working together to develop new diagnostic tools, therapeutic strategies, and preventive measures to improve patient outcomes and quality of life. Key areas of focus are:

Biomarker Discovery

Efforts are being made to identify biomarkers that can help with early detection, risk stratification, and monitoring of bowel obstruction. Researchers hope to develop non-invasive diagnostic tests that allow for early intervention and personalized management by identifying specific molecules or molecular signatures associated with obstruction.

Targeted Therapies

Researchers are looking into targeted therapeutic approaches that aim to address the root causes of bowel obstruction more precisely. These novel treatments, which range from molecularly targeted drugs to gene therapy and immunomodulatory agents, have the potential to improve efficacy while reducing side effects in comparison to conventional therapies.

Predictive Modeling

Advances in computational modeling and machine learning are being used to create predictive algorithms that can forecast the risk of bowel obstruction and guide treatment decisions. Researchers analyze large datasets of clinical and imaging data to identify patterns and predictors of obstruction recurrence, complications, and treatment response, allowing for more proactive and individualized care.

Regenerative Medicine

Regenerative medicine has the potential to repair damaged bowel tissue and restore normal function in patients suffering from obstructive disorders. Researchers are investigating a variety of approaches to promote tissue regeneration and repair defects in the gastrointestinal tract, including stem cell therapy, tissue engineering, and biomaterial scaffolds. These novel techniques present potential alternatives or adjuncts to traditional surgical interventions, to improve long-term outcomes and lower morbidity.

Hope For Patients And Families

Advances in bowel obstruction treatment, as well as ongoing research and innovation efforts, provide patients and their families with hope for better outcomes, a higher quality of life, and greater peace of mind. Healthcare providers are better prepared than ever to address the complex challenges posed by bowel obstruction, thanks to a multidisciplinary approach that combines medical expertise, technological innovation, and personalized care. By remaining at the forefront of research and embracing innovation, the future holds hope for better prospects and solutions for patients suffering from this condition.

CHAPTER 10

Living With Bowel Obstruction: Real Stories

Inspirational Stories Of Recovery

Despite the difficulties presented by intestinal blockage, many people have overcome hardship and made spectacular recoveries. Their experiences inspire and provide hope to those who are going through similar challenges.

Emily's tale is one such example since she was diagnosed with intestinal blockage at an early age. Despite having had several operations and medical procedures, Emily was determined to enjoy life to the fullest. Emily overcame the odds and regained her health because of her persistent dedication and cheerful outlook.

Another inspiring tale is that of Mark, who developed a passion for campaigning and awareness after being diagnosed with intestinal blockage. Mark utilized his experience to raise awareness about the disease and lobby for more resources and assistance for both patients and caretakers. His advocacy efforts not only assisted others suffering similar circumstances but also enabled him to discover purpose and meaning in his path.

Advice From Survivors And Caregivers

Navigating life with a bowel blockage may be difficult, but seeking counsel from survivors and caregivers who have been through this can offer vital direction and support.

One piece of advice often given by survivors is the need to advocate for oneself and obtain immediate medical assistance at the first indication of symptoms. Early management may dramatically improve results and avoid problems caused by intestinal blockage.

Caregivers often emphasize the necessity of self-care and request help from friends, family, and healthcare providers. Caregiving may be emotionally and physically taxing, and caregivers must prioritize their well-being to adequately assist their loved ones.

Furthermore, both survivors and caregivers stress the need to be educated about the disease and actively engage in treatment choices. Individuals who educate themselves about intestinal obstruction and its treatment might feel empowered to take an active part in their own or their loved one's care.

Finally, personal testimonies, inspiring tales of recovery, and guidance from survivors and caregivers provide essential insights and support to individuals living with intestinal blockage. Individuals may negotiate this road with strength, resilience, and optimism by sharing their stories, encouraging one another, and giving practical guidance.

CONCLUSION

Bowel blockage is a significant medical issue that needs immediate diagnosis and care to avert complications and protect the patient's well-being. The blockage may develop at any point along the gastrointestinal system, resulting in a variety of symptoms from minor discomfort to severe abdominal pain, vomiting, and constipation.

The diagnosis of intestinal blockage needs a complete medical history, physical examination, and several imaging investigations such as X-rays, CT scans, or ultrasound. Once identified, the therapy depends on the degree and source of the blockage.

Conservative therapy, including bowel rest, intravenous fluids, and nasogastric decompression, may be adequate for partial or simple blockages. However, full or complex blockages typically need surgical intervention to remove the blockage and ease symptoms.

The prognosis of intestinal blockage varies based on variables such as the underlying etiology, the timeliness of therapy, and the patient's general health state. While many instances may be effectively handled with proper medical or surgical intervention, delays in identification or treatment can lead to major consequences such as intestinal ischemia, perforation, or sepsis, which may dramatically impair patient outcomes.

In addition to medical therapy, patient education, and follow-up care are key parts of treating intestinal blockage. Patients should be instructed about dietary adjustments, lifestyle changes, and possible symptoms of problems to monitor for. Regular monitoring and contact with healthcare experts are critical for maintaining continuous treatment and avoiding recurrence.

Overall, early detection, timely management, and comprehensive treatment are crucial for maximizing outcomes in patients with intestinal blockage. Collaborative efforts between patients, healthcare professionals, and multidisciplinary teams are crucial in ensuring effective therapy and lowering the risk of complications associated with this illness.

THE END

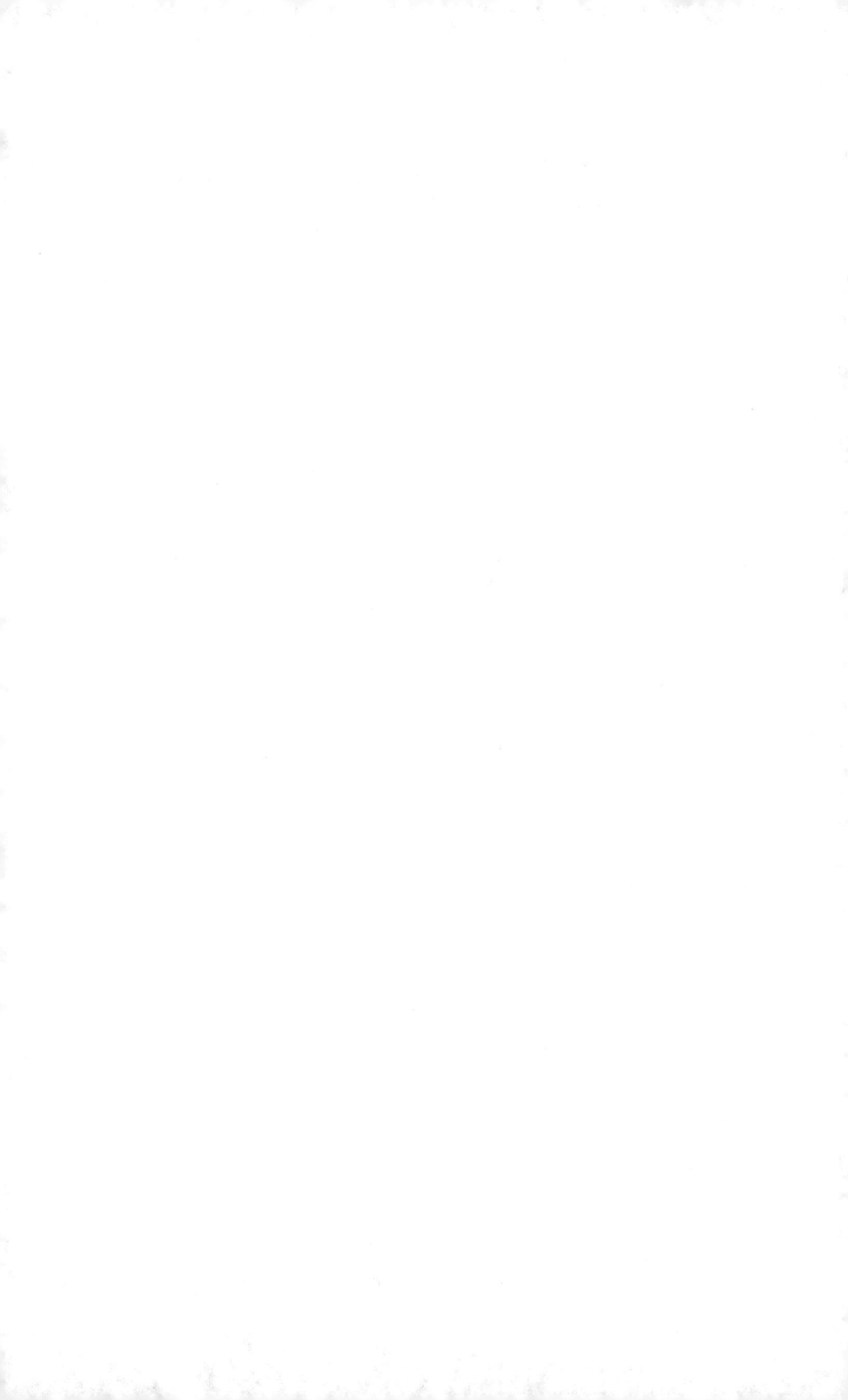

www.ingramcontent.com/pod-product-compliance
Lightning Source LLC
Chambersburg PA
CBHW050014230526
45470CB00003B/961